For Richard and William
as we watch you on your journey...

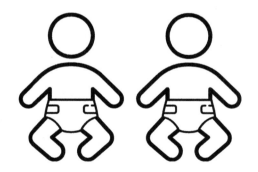

Contents:

So... How do you cope with your partner giving birth?

The truth is that we don't know...

This book was made to entertain you and your partner through a very exciting but challenging time in your lives. A novel way to keep conversation flowing whilst she's telling you to f*ck off.

Sometimes we all need a little laughter in moments of crisis. Some of us have the ability to find humour within us naturally, others need a little prompt... this book can do just that.

However, it's not all fun and games. We have also got a selection of challenging puzzles to go alongside all that laughter. Not to mention that we have been SUPER kind and included a glossary of key terms that crop up often when someone is giving birth.

Who knows... this book may even turn out to be useful?!

Disclaimer: *this book is a lot of nonsense, please dont hold us responsible for any of the facts here!*

Order of events checklist
Just to check you know how you got here...

We appreciate not everyone goes through these steps though...
Look at Jesus, he skipped to stage 3! Ultimately it doesn't matter how
you got here - getting to stage 4 is the important bit for you!

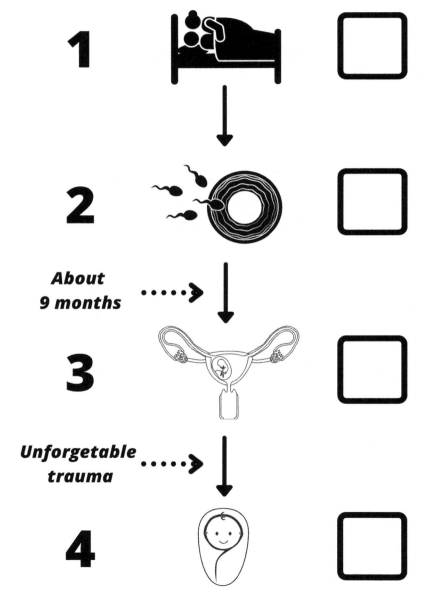

1

2

About 9 months ·····>

3

Unforgetable trauma ·····>

4

Some memes for you and the mum to be to get you started...

When my wife tells me she can feel the baby kicking

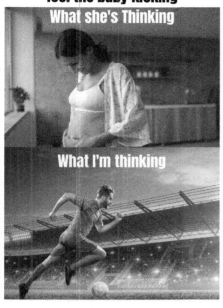

What she's Thinking

What I'm thinking

My wife when she is telling her friends that she thinks she has put on some extra baby weight and they agree

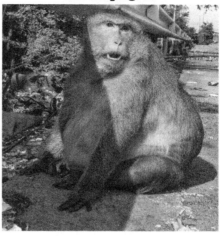

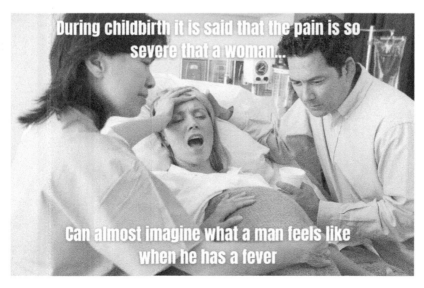

During childbirth it is said that the pain is so severe that a woman...

Can almost imagine what a man feels like when he has a fever

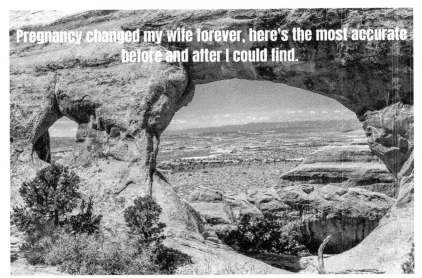

Pregnancy changed my wife forever, here's the most accurate before and after I could find.

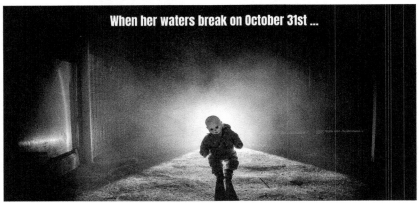

When her waters break on October 31st ...

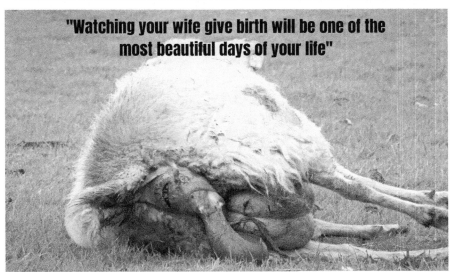

"Watching your wife give birth will be one of the most beautiful days of your life"

Crossword 1 - Pregnancy

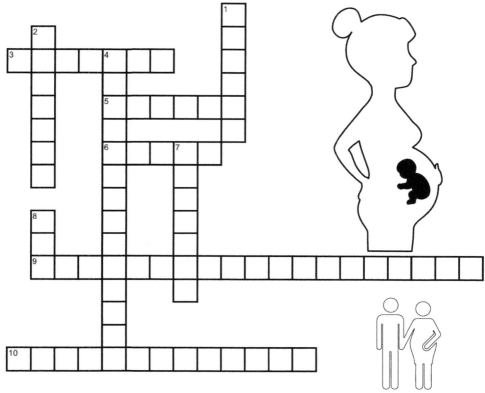

Across

3.What is the name of the health professional who will be looking after your partner and you baby? **(7)**

5.During the first 8 weeks of pregnancy the baby is referred to as what? **(6)**

6.How many months is each trimester of pregnancy? **(5)**

9.A problem that can result in the mother's blood sugar being too high. Sometimes the baby is also larger than usual? **(11, 8)**

10.This condition is commonly screened for between 10 and 14 weeks of pregnancy? **(5, 8)**

Down

1.Missing one of these may alert a woman to the fact she is pregnant? **(6)**

2.From how many weeks can your baby start hearing? **(7)**

4.What happens when a fertilised egg splits into two? **(8, 5)**

7.What do you call a pregnancy that implants in the Fallopian tube? **(7)**

8.A pregnancy test will come back positive if this hormone is present? **(3)**

Crossword 2 - Labour

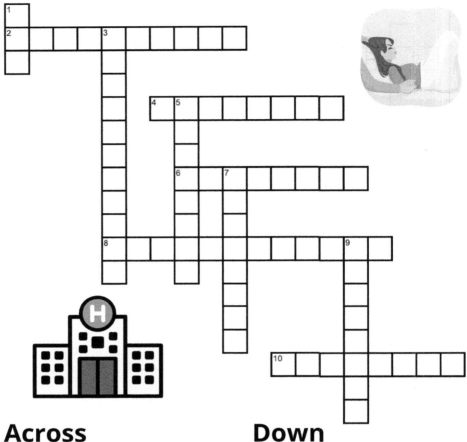

Across

2.The thinning and softening of the cervix is called? **(10)**

4.The pain relief that can be given by injection into the back? **(8)**

6.The term for when the baby's head starts to emerge? **(8)**

8.The type of doctor who may be involved in delivering the baby? **(12)**

10.The name of the suction cup instrument that may be used to help get the baby out? **(8)**

Down

1.The cervix is fully dilated at how many cm? **(3)**

3.The name of the cramping pain mothers may experience during labour? **(11)**

5.What is delivered in the third stage of labour? **(8)**

7.The name of the hormone that brings on contractions? **(8)**

9.The fluid sac that the baby is cased in? **(8)**

Crossword 3 - The Baby

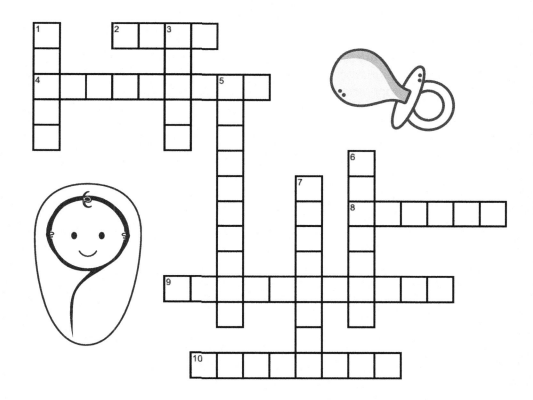

Across

2.Babies should sleep on their...? **(4)**

4.What term refers to a mothers sadness and low mood after giving birth? **(4,5)**

8.A common condition where babies bring back up their milk? **(6)**

9. The soft spots on the baby head are called? **(11)**

10.What is the first injection your newborn will receive? **(7,1)**

Down

1.With which part of your body should you check the temperature of a baby's bath? **(5)**

3.Excessive crying could mean your baby has this..although no-one knows what causes it? **(5)**

5.The process of squeezing milk out a mothers breast to store for later? **(10)**

6.The opposite of breast milk? **(7)**

7.The name of the first poo a baby passes? **(8)**

Trivia
Weird things people do with their placentas and umbilical cords

Many turn the placenta into pills and eat them... It is said that it reduces pain after birth, increases energy and helps breast milk but none of these are validated by any medical evidence!

Some (although we only found 1 report of this) mix it up their placenta with egg, sea salt and tannin and moulded the mixture into a teddy bear.

Some turn their placentas into art by using it to make a blood print. Some also use it to form a photo frame!

Some put the placenta in meals to make lasagne, chilli or even truffles!

BBQ placenta... Yes look it up online, it doesn't look too bad! Wear the placenta or umbilical cord as a necklace, or get it made into any jewellery you like.

Donate your umbilical cord and Save a life... The cord is rich in stem cells and can be used to treat diseases such as cancer, bone marrow failures, anaemias and many other disorders!

'Non-severance' this is when someone actually doesn't do anything to the placenta... Literally nothing. You simply carry it with you (sometimes referred to as a lotus bag).

Smoothies, Beauty treatment, Lip salve, Chocolate... At this point, you name it - it's probably been done!

True or False - Breastfeeding

Pick out the fact from the fiction

1. Exercise will affect the taste of milk   **TRUE** or **FALSE**

2. Breast feeding reduces the risk of ovarian cancer   **TRUE** or **FALSE**

3. The milk made in the first few days after birth is called colostrum   **TRUE** or **FALSE**

4. Bigger boobs produce more milk   **TRUE** or **FALSE**

5. Each nipple only has 1 milk opening   **TRUE** or **FALSE**

6. It's illegal to breastfeed in public   **TRUE** or **FALSE**

7. Breastfeeding reduces the chance of getting pregnant   **TRUE** or **FALSE**

8. Testosterone is responsible for milk production   **TRUE** or **FALSE**

9. Weaning is when solids are introduced into the baby's diet   **TRUE** or **FALSE**

10. High levels of caffeine should be avoided in breastfeeding. Chocolate contains caffeine   **TRUE** or **FALSE**

ANSWERS
1. FALSE 2. TRUE 3. TRUE 4. FALSE 5. FALSE
6. FALSE 7. TRUE 8. FALSE 9. TRUE 10. TRUE

True or False - Labour

Pick out the fact from the fiction

1. You can be in labour even if your water hasn't broken **TRUE** or **FALSE**

2. Sex and spicy foods will bring on labour **TRUE** or **FALSE**

3. You can be awake during a C-section **TRUE** or **FALSE**

4. Most babies are born on their due date? **TRUE** or **FALSE**

5. Having a 'show' or mucus plug means you're in labour **TRUE** or **FALSE**

6. Your birth plan must be stuck to **TRUE** or **FALSE**

7. Once you have a caesarean you can never have a vaginal birth **TRUE** or **FALSE**

8. Wide hips always make labour easier **TRUE** or **FALSE**

9. Skin to skin with the mother should be encouraged **TRUE** or **FALSE**

10. You can only give birth on your back **TRUE** or **FALSE**

True or False - General Pregnancy Myths

Pick out the fact from the fiction

1. Exercise is dangerous and should be avoided in pregnancy   **TRUE** or **FALSE**

2. A pregnant woman needs an extra 1000 calories a day   **TRUE** or **FALSE**

3. You shouldn't dye your hair   **TRUE** or **FALSE**

4. Morning sickness can happen any time of day   **TRUE** or **FALSE**

5. Babies can taste food you eat in the womb   **TRUE** or **FALSE**

6. Caffeine should be given up completely in pregnancy   **TRUE** or **FALSE**

7. Changing the cat litter is a safe activity?   **TRUE** or **FALSE**

8. Pregnancy causes your joints to loosen?   **TRUE** or **FALSE**

9. Morning sickness can predict the sex of the baby?   **TRUE** or **FALSE**

10. If a woman's hair is cut it could affect the baby's vision?   **TRUE** or **FALSE**

Baby names

Match the country to their most popular baby names! According to Wiki in 2021!

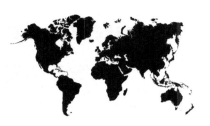

ASIA + OCEANIA

♂ **Oliver**	Malaysia
♀ **Isla**	New Zealand
♂ **Zhang Wei**	Pakistan
♂ **Haruto**	Turkey
♂ **Sky**	China
♀ **Nor**	Japan
♀ **Zeynep**	India
♀ **Fatima**	Australia

AFRICA

♂ **Mehdi**	Equatorial Guinea
♂ **Junior**	Tunisia
♂ **Mohamed**	Algeria
♀ **Fatoumata**	South Africa
♀ **Aya**	Libya
♀ **Imene**	Morocco
♂ **Manuel**	Egypt
♂ **Fatima**	Mali

Baby names

Match the country to their most popular baby names! According to Wiki in 2021!

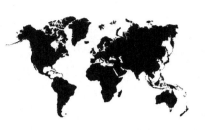

AMERICAS

♂ **Liam**	Argentina
♀ **Camila**	Venezuela
♂ **Ramón**	Greenland
♂ **Noah**	Brazil
♂ **Sebastián**	Puerto Rico
♀ **Ivaana**	USA
♀ **Maria**	Paraguay
♀ **Sofia**	Canada

EUROPE

♂ **Luka**	Netherlands
♂ **Daan**	Montenegro
♂ **Artem**	UK
♀ **Olivia**	Denmark
♀ **Ida**	Ukraine
♀ **Saga**	Finland
♂ **Dragan**	Serbia
♀ **Zala**	Slovenia

Multilingual babies

Here is a list of words that mean 'baby' all around the world... Can you match them up correctly?!
Join them up - we've done the easiest one!

Bebê	Brazilian
Beba	Czech
Nemluvñe	Croatian
Bebé	Spanish
Bébé	Finnish
Vauva	Japanese
赤ん坊	French
Dziecko	Polish
Bebeluș	Russian
Bebek	Turkish
Em bé	Vietnamese
ребенок	Romania
婴儿	Chinese
وَلِيد	English
Baby	Arabic

Wordsearch 1 - Labour

A	F	O	R	C	E	P	S	E	B	I	I	H	R
E	A	O	I	H	H	D	E	I	A	B	S	T	A
R	R	W	E	R	N	T	O	A	E	T	A	C	E
P	E	P	B	A	B	Y	A	O	E	A	D	S	E
H	C	E	E	R	B	P	U	B	U	E	I	O	B
R	H	S	U	P	E	U	R	R	R	C	O	S	N
H	N	A	E	R	A	S	E	A	C	E	W	R	M
W	U	H	E	P	I	D	U	R	A	L	T	S	I
B	L	O	O	D	S	W	O	O	A	O	U	A	D
N	O	I	T	C	A	R	T	N	O	C	A	C	W
E	U	W	I	S	A	N	I	E	R	T	O	S	I
O	L	A	R	T	U	T	E	R	U	S	H	B	F
B	T	P	L	A	C	E	N	T	A	I	B	D	E
U	O	A	A	N	A	D	O	I	P	U	L	C	P

BREECH	UTERUS
CONTRACTION	BLOOD
BABY	CAESAREAN
FORCEPS	PUSH
WATERBATH	PLACENTA
EPIDURAL	MIDWIFE

Wordsearch 2 - The Baby

M	U	S	L	I	N	I	C	M	C	U	O	O	L
N	T	V	E	B	T	O	E	I	B	U	U	C	N
N	A	A	E	R	A	U	O	L	A	E	G	A	K
A	N	C	A	E	L	M	N	K	G	O	T	L	A
P	D	C	K	A	C	T	E	E	T	H	I	N	G
P	N	I	O	S	U	R	D	U	M	M	Y	F	Y
Y	N	N	O	T	M	C	B	O	T	W	B	O	E
D	D	A	B	F	P	M	M	C	R	Y	I	N	G
N	D	T	D	E	O	M	I	U	C	U	G	S	P
I	M	I	E	E	W	I	T	M	A	R	N	H	G
C	P	O	R	D	D	E	T	P	L	L	D	G	N
R	O	N	I	I	E	T	I	I	P	E	S	I	P
G	R	S	T	N	R	M	M	K	O	G	I	T	S
I	D	M	E	G	M	D	L	I	L	T	M	V	Y

BREASTFEEDING   MILK

TIRED   MUSLIN

CRYING   TEETHING

TALCUM POWDER   VACCINATIONS

CALPOL   NAPPY

DUMMY   RED BOOK

Wordsearch 3 - Pregnancy

A	N	T	E	N	A	T	A	L	C	L	A	S	S
M	O	T	C	U	S	I	L	I	S	H	T	D	B
O	R	D	N	U	O	S	A	R	T	L	U	M	U
O	T	A	R	E	I	I	Y	I	E	G	T	S	M
D	O	E	S	M	O	M	D	G	A	R	I	C	P
S	N	Y	S	T	N	T	R	O	R	E	F	R	O
W	O	U	G	N	S	F	T	N	E	N	E	I	D
I	C	F	O	L	I	C	A	C	I	D	R	C	N
N	D	P	S	A	M	E	F	C	L	N	T	W	H
G	F	S	C	R	E	E	N	I	N	G	G	F	A
S	O	E	T	R	T	R	I	M	E	S	T	E	R
M	R	O	H	E	A	R	T	B	U	R	N	E	B
C	O	N	O	Y	R	B	M	E	E	T	I	C	B
E	N	N	S	S	G	N	I	V	A	R	C	E	R

TRIMESTER   HEARTBURN

SCREENING   ANTENATAL CLASS

MOOD SWINGS   CRAVINGS

FOLIC ACID   EMBRYO

BUMP   ULTRASOUND

Wordsearch 4 - What's in the bag?

T	A	L	M	I	L	K	B	O	T	T	L	E	G
N	I	S	E	P	I	W	T	E	W	C	S	H	A
K	B	L	A	N	K	E	T	T	H	N	T	A	M
A	I	E	I	K	E	P	B	A	O	A	S	N	P
M	G	T	S	N	A	T	N	P	I	E	N	D	A
U	I	E	I	C	N	G	I	L	N	W	A	S	C
S	L	M	I	B	I	E	T	A	T	S	P	A	I
L	C	L	E	N	E	P	S	S	M	N	P	N	F
I	R	N	G	E	I	S	E	T	E	S	Y	I	I
N	O	M	T	I	F	H	I	I	N	W	T	T	E
A	A	I	I	E	T	N	L	C	T	N	S	I	R
T	S	M	I	O	C	T	O	B	O	H	P	S	O
S	S	H	L	W	E	E	P	A	Y	M	I	E	L
P	A	C	W	S	G	F	E	G	S	W	I	R	T

CLOTHES
WET WIPES
CHANGING MAT
OINTMENT
NAPPY
HAND SANITISER

MUSLIN
TOYS
PLASTIC BAG
MILK BOTTLE
PACIFIER
BLANKET

Atypical name generator

BABY BOY ♂

First Name: 3rd Letter of your First name	Middle name: Last letter of your 2nd name
A - Ezra	A - Keir
B - Rex	B - Che
C - Tyson	C - Lion
D - Ace	D - Remus
E - Pax	E - Albus
F - Cruze	F - Aragon
G - Pepper	G - Octavius
H - Mars	H - Ziggy
I - Gary	I - Knox
J - Fenton	J - Walt
K - Duke	K - Dewey
L - Heston	L - Zarel
M - Sherlock	M - Jethro
N - Blaze	N - Otto
O - Kaya	O - Titus
P - Thane	P - Adonis
Q - Ace	Q - Jetaime
R - Cynan	R - Danyon
S - Rafe	S - Drey
T - Zeus	T - Zephyr
U - Sergio	U- Bear
V - Malakai	V - Ryker
W - Tahir	W - Neo
X - Tarquin	X - Huxley
Y - Rico	Y - Legend
Z - Wolf	Z - Kenzo

BABY GIRL ♀

First Name: First letter of your first name	Middle name: 2nd letter your 2nd name
A - Luna	A - Khaleesi
B - Lyra	B - Skyla
C - Nova	C - Moana
D - Juniper	D - Jubilee
E - Mila	E - Ripley
F - Noa	F - Halo
G - Elowen	G - Honesty
H - Arya	H - Egypt
I - Daenerys	I - Whimsey
J - Soleil	J - Aubrielle
K - Rue	K - Bristol
L - Alpen	L - Charleigh
M - Aldonna	M - Blessing
N - Bellamy	N - Maybelle
O - Navy	O - Eleven
P - Heaven	P - Genesis
Q - Maple	Q - Hermoine
R - Holland	R - Pertunia
S - Story	S - Jessa
T - Kehlani	T - Laken
U - Zendaya	U - Zoya
V - Capri	V - Vanellope
W - Lyric	W - Sisa
X - Alivia	X - True
Y - Pixie	Y - Zhavia
Z - Snow	Z - Anniston

Jokes for the big day
(Appropriate)

What do a pregnancy test and hummus have in common? They both require chickpea...

I recently learned that goats can have what's called a "phantom pregnancy." It's when their body thinks it's pregnant when it isn't. I kid you not.

This pregnancy test I just took confirmed my worst fear. I'm just fat.

I once told story about pregnancy that nobody understood except for my twin sister - It was our little inside joke

I have this app idea, it's a pregnancy test. You piss on the phone, and if the phone is covered in piss you're not allowed to have kids.

When answering the security question place of birth... Apparently vagina is not an acceptable answer!

What form of birth control works better with holes in it? Crocs

Do I have to have a baby shower?
Not if you change the baby's nappy very quickly...

Jokes for the big day
(Inappropriate)

Success is like pregnancy.
Everybody congratulates you but nobody knows how many times you got f*cked to achieve it.

Why was Hitler's mum so happy during her entire pregnancy?
Because she had a dick inside her for 9 months

The stork is the bird that helps deliver babies. What bird helps prevent pregnancy? The swallow.

"How did the blind girl explain her pregnancy?"
She said she didn't see him coming

Had to get castrated today for birth control reasons.
I paid so much and they didn't even use scissors.
It was a rip-off.

Our doctor told us we could have sex right up until the time of the baby's birth... I don't know why they got so upset with me in the delivery room?!

How do you get a nun pregnant?
Dress her up as an altar boy.

Everything is made in China... Except for baby girls

Jokes for the big day
(The Dad joke specials)

I bought a home pregnancy kit... Turns out my house is pregnant.

A woman covered in pasta sauce takes a pregnancy test. Turns out she's Prego

Never talk to a girl about pregnancy, periods or 'women problems' ... She'll ovary act

What do you call it when someone's unable to find someone able to help them through their pregnancy? Having a midwife crisis

Scientists have found that sunblock is actually 50% effective as birth control... Because it only blocks the sons

How do mermaids give birth?
They get a sea-section.

How warm is a baby at birth? Womb temperature.

A woman in England gives birth every 30 seconds. She must be exhausted!

Bingo Time

Things you hear!

"You have no Idea how I feel!"	"Get a towel!"	"I can see the head!"
"You're fully dilated!"	"PUSH"	"I can't do this!"
"SQUEEZE!"	"F*CK/ F*CK OFF/ OH MY F*CK"	"Deep Breaths!"

Bingo Time

Things you see!

Baby's Head	Poo	Entonox (Gas and air)
A ridiculous birthing position	Forceps	Umbilical Cord
A midwife running	Blood	A Doctor

Glossary of terms (1/4)

Amniotic fluid: Sometimes called liquor, this is the fluid that surrounds the baby in the uterus (womb).

Amniotic sac: The bag in which the fetus and amniotic fluid are contained during pregnancy.

Antenatal: Before the birth.

Antepartum haemorrhage (APH): Bleeding before the birth.

Assisted delivery: The use of forceps or ventouse to speed up the delivery, or to move the baby if they have become stuck.

Breech presentation: This means your baby is lying bottom or feet down in the uterus.

Blood pressure (BP): It's important to have your blood pressure measured as a rise could mean a problem.

Caesarean section: Delivery of an infant through an incision in the abdominal and uterine walls.

Congenital: Present at birth.

Crowning: The point in labour when the head of the baby can be seen at the vagina.

Dilation/Dilatation: In the first stage of labour the cervix, or neck of the womb, gradually opens up to make space for the baby. It needs to open to approximately 10 centimetres before the baby's head can pass through. This process is called dilation of the cervix.

Eclampsia: A serious complication of pregnancy, characterised by high blood pressure and oedema (swelling), which in its worse form can result in a seizure (fit). It is the more severe form of pre-eclampsia.

Ectopic Pregnancy: A pregnancy that develops somewhere other than the uterus, usually in the fallopian tube. This pregnancy cannot be allowed to continue as it is dangerous.

Engaged: This means that the widest part of the baby's head has passed into the pelvis in preparation for giving birth.

Entonox: A mixture of oxygen and nitrous oxide, inhaled through a mask or mouthpiece by the mother during labour for pain relief. Also called gas and air or gas and oxygen.

Epidural: An injection of local anaesthetic into the lower back, given for pain relief during labour. This can be topped up via a catheter (a thin tube) that is left in place during labour. For most women an epidural takes away all the pain of contractions.

Episiotomy: A cut made in the mother's perineum (the area between the vagina and anus) to allow the baby to be born more quickly and prevent tearing.

Fetus: Medical name for the baby before it's born.

Glossary of terms (2/4)

Fetal Movement (FM): It may say 'FM felt' or 'FMF' on your notes. That means your baby had been felt to move.

First stage of labour: The time from the beginning of labour until the cervix is fully dilated to 10cm. The first stage can vary from a few hours to 12 hours or more.

FML (F*ck my life): Usually said during a negative experience.

Fontanelles: The two soft spots on a newborn's head where the skull bones do not yet meet.

Forceps: A pair of hollow blades, rather like large salad servers, which are placed either side of the baby's head to assist with the birth. When this happens, it is known as a forceps delivery.

Fundus: This is the top of the uterus. The 'fundal' height helps assess the growth of the baby and how many weeks pregnant you are. It's the length in centimetres between the top of the uterus and the pubic bone.

Gestation/Gestational age: How far into the pregnancy you are, measured from the first day of your last menstrual period.

Haemorrhage: Sudden and severe bleeding. In pregnancy it is usually called antepartum haemorrhage and after the birth it is called postpartum haemorrhage. Any bleeding in pregnancy should be reported to a doctor or midwife.

Hyper/hypotension: High/low blood pressure.

Induction: Starting the labour artificially.

Latent phase of labour: Also known as early labour. This is when a woman starts to experience contractions, which which can be irregular in strength and frequency and can last from a few hours to several days. Some women will also experience backache. The contractions will, over a period of time, usually increase in strength and frequency until they cause your cervix (the neck of the womb) to dilate. Once the cervix is 4cm dilated the labour is said to have become established and the active phase commences.

Meconium: The bowel contents of the baby at birth.

Membrane sweep: A traditional method of trying to nudge the body into labour when overdue. The doctor or midwife does an internal examination and attempts to stretch the cervix and sweep a finger around the membranes. Sometimes this is enough to get labour going if the cervix is ripe.

Multigravida: A woman who has been pregnant before.

Multipara: Also called a multip – a woman who has given birth at least once before.

Neonate: A newborn infant.

Glossary of terms (3/4)

Obstetrician: A doctor who specialises in the care of women during pregnancy and childbirth.

Occipito Anterior: When the back of your baby's head is toward your front. You may see LOA or ROA on your notes which means Left (or Right) occipito anterior and described whether the baby's head is toward the left or the right. LOA is usually the best position for a shorter labour and an easier birth.

Occipito Posterior: As above but the baby's head is toward your back.

Oxytocin: The hormone secreted by women when they are in labour which stimulates labour contractions. The same hormone also stimulates milk flow from the breasts by contracting the muscle fibres in the milk ducts.

Postnatal: After the birth. Relates to the 28 day period following giving birth.

Postpartum: Relating to the period of a few days after the birth.

Pre-eclampsia: This is a complication of pregnancy where the blood pressure increases and protein appears in the urine.

Pregnancy Induced Hypertension: This means that your blood pressure is high a result of the pregnancy.

Presentation: The part of the baby which is coming first (usually the crown or back of the baby's head).

Preterm: Born before 37 weeks of pregnancy.

Primigravida: A woman pregnant for the first time.

Primipara: Sometimes called the prim or primip – a woman giving birth for the first time.

Prolapsed umbilical cord: Usually the baby's cord is born along with the baby and it continues to supply oxygen to the baby until it is clamped and cut. Occasionally the cord slips down in front of the baby and the oxygen supply to the baby is reduced or cut off. This can happen with a breech baby or with a transverse or unstable lie. This is a medical emergency and the baby has be delivered very quickly, usually by an emergency Caesarean section.

Prostaglandin: A natural substance used in pessaries to soften the cervix and stimulate the start of labour.

Pudendal block: A local anaesthetic given to block pain around the cervix and vagina before using forceps.

Rhesus (Rh): The rhesus blood group system is a way of categorising your blood type.

Second stage of labour: The time from full dilation of the cervix to the moment when the baby is outside the mother's body. Pushing during the second stage can last from a few minutes up to a couple of hours. Show: A show is when the thick mucus which plugs the narrow channel of the cervix during pregnancy comes away. It is a sign that the body is getting ready for labour.

Glossary of terms (4/4)

Skin-to-skin: Skin-to-skin contact with your baby after birth (your baby is dried and put straight onto your chest).

Syntocinon: This is a synthetic version of a naturally made hormone called oxytocin which increases contractions. It is sometimes used to speed up labours that have become slow, or to reduce bleeding after a baby is born. It is also sometimes given to speed up the delivery of the placenta. It is always given as an injection, either into a muscle or vein.

Syntometrine: This contains two drugs (syntocinon and ergomerine) that help the womb contract after the baby is born. It is sometimes used to speed up the delivery of the placenta or to stop bleeding after birth.

TENS: Transcutaneous Electrical Nerve Stimulation – a device for relieving the pain of labour. Sticky pads are attached to the woman's back to produce electrical impulses which stimulate her own natural painkillers and block some of the pain signals from the uterus. The unit is battery operated and the woman can control the amount of stimulation herself with a push button device and a variable control dial.

Term: This used to describe the period of time at the end of a pregnancy when a baby might be expected to be born. It is 37-42 weeks which is the normal duration of a human pregnancy.

Third stage: Delivery of the placenta (afterbirth).

Transition: The tough-going, final part of the first stage of labour, when the mother may begin to feel the urge to push. Contractions may come thick and fast and can feel very hard to cope with.

Transverse lie: A baby who is lying across the uterus horizontally, rather than vertically. In this position the baby cannot be born and there is a high risk of the cord prolapsing.

Trimester: One third of a pregnancy.

Ultrasound scan: A screening or diagnostic technique in which very high frequency sound waves are passed into the body, and the reflected echoes are detected and analysed to build a picture of the internal organs or of a fetus in the uterus.

Umbilical cord: The thick cord of intertwining blood vessels that links baby and placenta, and carries oxygen and nourishment to the baby.

Unstable lie: The baby changes position often and cannot be considered to be in any definite position.

Uterus or womb: The hollow muscular organ in which the baby lives until birth.

Ventouse: This is the name given to a method of vacuum extraction to help the baby be born at the end of the labour, either if the mother is very tired or if the baby has become distressed.

Answers

Crossword 1: Pregnancy

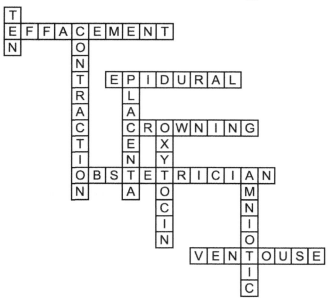

Crossword 2: Labour

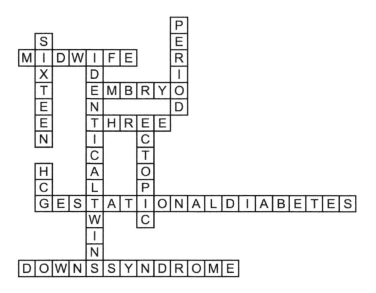

Answers
Crossword 3: The Baby

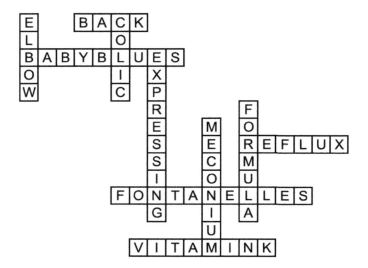

Answers
Wordsearches (1/2)

DURING LABOUR

A	F	O	R	C	E	P	S	E	B	I	I	H	R
E	A	O	I	H	H	D	E	I	A	B	S	T	A
R	R	W	E	R	N	T	O	A	E	T	A	C	E
P	E	P	B	A	B	Y	A	O	E	A	D	S	E
H	C	E	E	R	B	P	U	B	U	E	I	O	B
R	H	S	U	P	E	U	R	R	R	C	O	S	N
H	N	A	E	R	A	S	E	A	C	E	W	R	M
W	U	H	E	P	I	D	U	R	A	L	T	S	I
B	L	O	O	D	S	W	O	O	A	O	U	A	D
N	O	I	T	C	A	R	T	N	O	C	A	C	W
E	U	W	I	S	A	N	I	E	R	T	O	S	I
O	L	A	R	T	U	T	E	R	U	S	H	B	F
B	T	P	L	A	C	E	N	T	A	I	B	D	E
U	O	A	A	N	A	D	O	I	P	U	L	C	P

BREECH
CONTRACTION
BABY
FORCEPS
WATERBATH
EPIDURAL
UTERUS
BLOOD
CAESAREAN
PUSH
PLACENTA
MIDWIFE

THE BABY IS HERE!

M	U	S	L	I	N	I	C	M	C	U	O	O	L
N	T	V	E	B	T	O	E	I	B	U	U	C	N
N	A	A	E	R	A	U	O	L	A	E	G	A	K
A	N	C	A	E	L	M	N	K	G	O	T	L	A
P	D	C	K	A	C	T	E	E	T	H	I	N	G
P	N	I	O	S	U	R	D	U	M	M	Y	F	Y
Y	N	N	O	T	M	C	B	O	T	W	B	O	E
D	D	A	B	F	P	M	M	C	R	Y	I	N	G
N	D	T	D	E	O	M	I	U	C	U	G	S	P
I	M	I	E	E	W	I	T	M	A	R	N	H	G
C	P	O	R	D	D	E	T	P	L	L	D	G	N
R	O	N	I	I	E	T	I	I	P	E	S	I	P
G	R	S	T	N	R	M	M	K	O	G	I	T	S
I	D	M	E	G	M	D	L	I	L	T	M	V	Y

BREASTFEEDING
TIRED
CRYING
TALCUM POWDER
CALPOL
DUMMY
MILK
MUSLIN
TEETHING
VACCINATIONS
NAPPY
RED BOOK

Answers
Wordsearches (2/2)

LOOKING BACK ON PREGNANCY

A	N	T	E	N	A	T	A	L	C	L	A	S	S
M	O	T	C	U	S	I	L	I	S	H	T	D	B
O	R	D	N	U	O	S	A	R	T	L	U	M	U
O	T	A	R	E	I	I	Y	I	E	G	T	S	M
D	O	E	S	M	O	M	D	G	A	R	I	C	P
S	N	Y	S	T	N	T	R	O	R	E	F	R	O
W	O	U	G	N	S	F	T	N	E	N	E	I	D
I	C	F	O	L	I	C	A	C	I	D	R	C	N
N	D	P	S	A	M	E	F	C	L	N	T	W	H
G	F	S	C	R	E	E	N	I	N	G	G	F	A
S	O	E	T	R	T	R	I	M	E	S	T	E	R
M	R	O	H	E	A	R	T	B	U	R	N	E	B
C	O	N	O	Y	R	B	M	E	E	T	I	C	B
E	N	N	S	S	G	N	I	V	A	R	C	E	R

TRIMESTER
SCREENING
MOOD SWINGS
FOLIC ACID
BUMP
HEARTBURN
ANTENATAL CLASS
CRAVINGS
EMBRYO
ULTRASOUND

THINGS TO HAVE IN YOUR BAG...

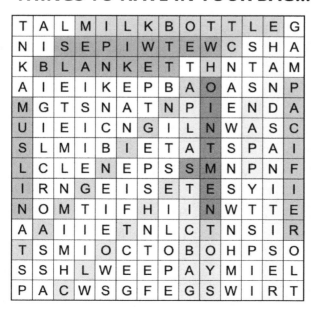

T	A	L	M	I	L	K	B	O	T	T	L	E	G
N	I	S	E	P	I	W	T	E	W	C	S	H	A
K	B	L	A	N	K	E	T	T	H	N	T	A	M
A	I	E	I	K	E	P	B	A	O	A	S	N	P
M	G	T	S	N	A	T	N	P	I	E	N	D	A
U	I	E	I	C	N	G	I	L	N	W	A	S	C
S	L	M	I	B	I	E	T	A	T	S	P	A	I
L	C	L	E	N	E	P	S	S	M	N	P	N	F
I	R	N	G	E	I	S	E	T	E	S	Y	I	I
N	O	M	T	I	F	H	I	I	N	W	T	T	E
A	A	I	I	E	T	N	L	C	T	N	S	I	R
T	S	M	I	O	C	T	O	B	O	H	P	S	O
S	S	H	L	W	E	E	P	A	Y	M	I	E	L
P	A	C	W	S	G	F	E	G	S	W	I	R	T

CLOTHES
WET WIPES
CHANGING MAT
OINTMENT
NAPPY
HAND SANITISER
MUSLIN
TOYS
PLASTIC BAG
MILK BOTTLE
PACIFIER
BLANKET

Answers - Baby names

ASIA + OCEANA

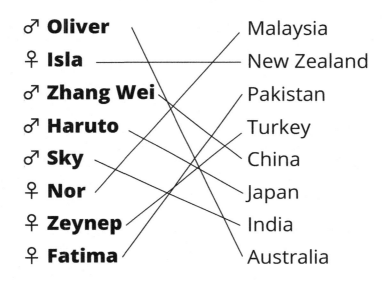

♂ Oliver	Malaysia
♀ Isla	New Zealand
♂ Zhang Wei	Pakistan
♂ Haruto	Turkey
♂ Sky	China
♀ Nor	Japan
♀ Zeynep	India
♀ Fatima	Australia

AFRICA

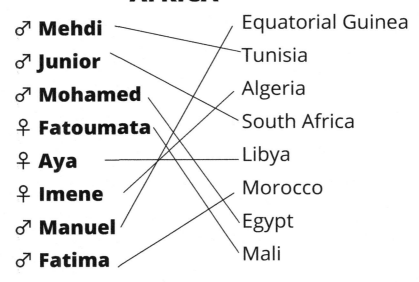

♂ Mehdi	Equatorial Guinea
♂ Junior	Tunisia
♂ Mohamed	Algeria
♀ Fatoumata	South Africa
♀ Aya	Libya
♀ Imene	Morocco
♂ Manuel	Egypt
♂ Fatima	Mali

Answers - Baby names

AMERICAS

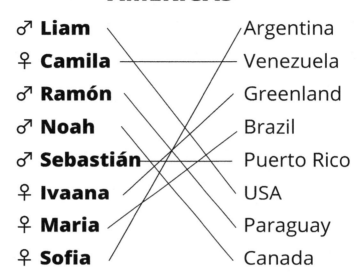

♂ **Liam** — USA

♀ **Camila** — Paraguay

♂ **Ramón** — Puerto Rico

♂ **Noah** — Greenland

♂ **Sebastián** — Venezuela

♀ **Ivaana** — Canada

♀ **Maria** — Brazil

♀ **Sofia** — Argentina

EUROPE

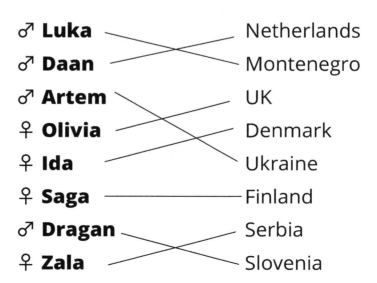

♂ **Luka** — Montenegro

♂ **Daan** — Netherlands

♂ **Artem** — Denmark

♀ **Olivia** — UK

♀ **Ida** — Ukraine

♀ **Saga** — Finland

♂ **Dragan** — Slovenia

♀ **Zala** — Serbia

Answers - Multilingual

Bebê —————— Brazilian

Beba ⟍   ⟋ Czech

Nemluvñe ⟍⟋ Croatian

Bebé —————— Spanish

Bébé ⟍   ⟋ Finnish

Vauva ⟋⟍ Japanese

赤ん坊 ⟋   ⟍ French

Dziecko —————— Polish

Bebeluș ⟍ Russian

Bebek ⟋⟍ Turkish

Em bé ⟋⟍ Vietnamese

ребенок ⟋   ⟍ Romania

婴儿 —————— Chinese

وَليد ⟍   ⟋ English

Baby ⟋⟍ Arabic

THE END

Alas, it is just the beginning for you and your new life...

We hope this book provided some light relief during a very stressful time.

Don't forget to remind your birthing partner that whilst she had to endure *some* pain in the process of childbirth **YOU** were the one who had to stand up and watch the whole thing... Like going to a cinema and watching the worst horror film of all time, on your feet and without the popcorn.

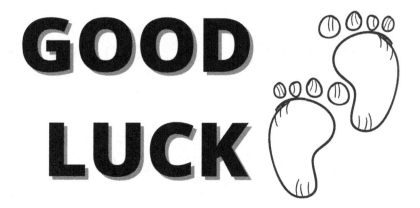

GOOD LUCK